Diets to help
CANDIDA

Also in this series:

DIETS TO HELP ARTHRITIS
Helen MacFarlane

DIETS TO HELP ASTHMA AND HAY FEVER
Roger Newman Turner

DIETS TO HELP COLITIS AND IBS
Joan Lay

DIETS TO HELP CONTROL CHOLESTEROL
Roger Newman Turner

DIETS TO HELP CYSTITIS
Ralph McCutcheon

DIETS TO HELP DIABETES
Martin Budd

DIETS TO HELP GLUTEN AND WHEAT ALLERGY
Rita Greer

DIETS TO HELP MULTIPLE SCLEROSIS
Rita Greer

DIETS TO HELP PSORIASIS
Harry Clements

Diets to help
CANDIDA

LEON CHAITOW

Thorsons
An Imprint of HarperCollinsPublishers

Thorsons
An Imprint of HarperCollins*Publishers*
77–85 Fulham Palace Road,
Hammersmith, London W6 8JB
1160 Battery Street
San Francisco, California 94111–1213

First published 1997
10 9 8 7 6 5 4 3 2

A catalogue record for this book
is available from the British Library

ISBN 0 7225 3423 X

Printed and bound in Great Britain by
Caledonian International Book Manufacturing Ltd, Glasgow

Contents

The recipes and general food preparation tips found in later chapters of this book owe much to the ideas of my wife, Alkmini, whose excellent book *Greek Vegetarian Cooking* (Thorsons) was an inspiration for much of the information. For this and her support during the writing of the book, I dedicate it to her with my profound thanks.

Introduction

Candida albicans is a yeast which lives in all of us, usually confined to tiny colonies in the lower end of the digestive tract, the vagina and certain skin areas. This yeast is usually controlled by our defence (immune) systems, as well as by a host of friendly bacteria with which we enjoy a symbiotic relationship (we benefit and they benefit) and which live in large numbers in our digestive tracts. They are provided with both food and lodging, in return for which they perform certain vital roles, including manufacturing some of the B-vitamins, detoxifying the bowel, recycling various important substances such as oestrogen and cholesterol and – most important – keeping undesirable alien bacteria and yeasts out of the digestive tract. The most prominent of the friendly bacteria are acidophilus, which lives in the small intestine, and bifidobacteria, which lives in the colon.

WHY CANDIDA ACTIVITY INCREASES

When our diet is very sugary or contains excessive amounts of fat, the friendly bacteria become less efficient in performing the many vital functions which are helpful to us. They are also adversely affected when we take certain medication. In particular, the use of antibiotics and steroid medication (including the contraceptive pill) can be severely damaging to them. A possible consequence of their impaired functioning is the spread of yeasts, such as Candida, further into the intestinal tract, and sometimes into the body generally.

Candida albicans, which is best known for causing thrush in the mouth or the vagina, is found in two forms, as a simple yeast and also as a damaging fungus which puts down 'rootlets' (rhizomes) into the smooth inner surface of the intestinal tract, the mucous membrane. This transformation, from yeast to an aggressive fungus, occurs when the natural control mechanisms exerted by the friendly bacteria are weakened. One particularly important element of this control is Biotin – one of the B-vitamins – which is manufactured by the intestinal flora and which prevents yeast from turning into its aggressive form. If Biotin is deficient and yeast becomes a mycelial fungus, the consequent damage to the protective mucous membrane allows undesirable toxins to permeate into the bloodstream. This condition, often called 'leaky gut' syndrome, is highly likely to lead to allergic reactions which are reflected in the development of many symptoms.

SYMPTOMS OF CANDIDA ACTIVITY

Among the many symptoms recorded in people affected in this way, especially if their diet is sugar-rich, are a
range of digestive problems (bloating and irritable
bowel, in which there are recurrent episodes of either
diarrhoea or constipation), urinary tract infections,
menstrual disturbances, extreme fatigue, muscle aches,
emotional disturbances, 'foggy' brain syndrome and
skin problems. The frequency with which such symptoms are suffered by many people is staggering.

Amongst the most persistent symptoms, apart from
those affecting the digestive tract, are chronic fatigue
and chronic muscle pain. Those recorded by just one
medical expert can help us to see the range of problems
hiding behind this yeast.

Dr Carol Jessop, an internal medicine specialist from
San Francisco, presented details of over 1,300 of her
patients with chronic fatigue and muscle pain
(fibromyalgia) to a 1990 medical symposium in
Charlotte, North Carolina. She reported that nearly 90
per cent of them (both men and women) had yeast
infections and that the vast majority of these had
records of frequent and recurrent antibiotic use for
sinus, acne, prostate, urinary tract and chest infections
in the main. Of the women, 70 per cent with chronic
fatigue and/or muscle pain had been on 'the pill' for
three years or more and 63 per cent reported a sugar
craving.

TESTS?

A history of antibiotic use in anything other than isolated and brief instances, a high sugar diet and/or the use of steroid medication are the chief clues, yet even so expensive laboratory tests for the presence of yeast are commonly inaccurate. Why should this be so?

Because yeast lives in and on all of us, it may be found even when there is no actual health problem associated with its presence. On the other hand, and quite surprisingly, even when it is widely active in areas where it is normally controlled it is often difficult to detect using standard tests.

One of the most effective tests uses 'sugar loading' or gut fermentation. This involves the subject swallowing a set amount of pure sugar on an empty stomach after a sample of blood has been taken. A second sample is taken an hour later and the level of alcohol in the blood, before and after the sugar intake, is measured. Because yeast – and some bacteria – can turn sugar into alcohol rapidly in the intestines, a rise in blood alcohol is used as a diagnostic sign. However, because this can also occur through bacterial overgrowth in the intestines it does not prove yeast is the culprit.

World renowned experts in the study of the ill-effects of Candida on people's health – such as the American physician William Crook – now rely on a simple questionnaire (current symptoms, health history and previous use of antibiotics and steroid medication) to indicate the possibility, probability or slight chance of yeast being a part of the person's health problems.

TREATMENT

Medical care of Candida problems such as thrush usually focuses on the local outbreak – most commonly in the mouth or vagina. This sort of treatment may well get rid of local symptoms for a short time, but it fails to address the fact that in almost all cases of obvious yeast infection (such as thrush) there is a 'reservoir' of yeast activity in the digestive tract which has to be controlled or eliminated if the thrush (or other local infection) is not to return every few weeks or months.

Even when systemic or digestive tract Candida (or other yeast) infection is dealt with by medical drugs there is seldom any attempt at repopulation of the tract with friendly bacterial colonies, or of any dietary modification to support the anti-yeast programme. This means that more often than not medical anti-Candida methods have only limited success.

The most effective method of getting yeast under control (we never completely eliminate it since it is a 'normal' inhabitant of everyone) involves a combined strategy which:

- Deprives yeast of its main nutrient – sugar.
- Eliminates from the diet (for a while) yeast-based or yeast-containing substances and foods, since there is a strong likelihood that anyone with a Candida problem will have become sensitized to yeast and its by-products.

- Kills the yeast – and a wide range of common foods and substances, including garlic and olive oil, can help in this work.
- Repopulates the intestinal tract with healthy friendly bacterial colonies (acidophilus and bifidobacteria).
- Gives general immune system support by ensuring a balanced wholesome, nutritious diet.

My book *Candida Albicans – Could Yeast be Your Problem?* (Thorsons) gives full details of this combined approach, while this book provides comprehensive advice on constructing a dietary pattern which will support recovery from yeast infection.

CHAPTER ONE

Cutting Sugar to Conquer Candida

Yeast loves sugar – ask any wine or beer maker! Candida thrives on sugar and all refined carbohydrates. It also benefits from anything which increases your blood-sugar levels, such as adrenaline-releasing stimulants – tea, coffee, chocolate, alcohol, cigarettes and, of course, stress.

A low-sugar diet, therefore, means more than just cutting down the obvious sugars – it also means finding substitutes for the regularly consumed stimulants – and it calls for you to begin to relax and to adopt stress-coping strategies (sufficient rest, a calmer attitude, relaxation and meditation, more sleep and adequate exercise).

In the early stages of any anti-Candida diet (three to four weeks) it is also wise to reduce all fruit intake and, for the duration (up to six months), to avoid fruit drinks (bottled, fresh, canned, frozen) and very sweet fruits (melons, grapes, etc.) since these rapidly increase blood sugar levels.

Refined carbohydrates (white flour and its products, for example) are equally undesirable and should be eliminated during the programme. Many experts suggest that milk sugar (lactose) should also be avoided until yeast is well and truly under control, and in any case for the first three to four weeks of any anti-Candida effort.

All canned and frozen and packaged foods should be examined for their contents, and the following should be avoided completely: fructose, glucose, glycogen, galactose, lactose, maltose, mannitol, monosaccharides, polysaccharides, sorbitol and sucrose.

For the entire period of an anti-Candida diet you should avoid all forms of obvious sweetening, such as sugar (any colour), honey, molasses, maple syrup and date sugar, as well as dried fruits (all), malt extracts and products and alcoholic beverages of all sorts.

Be very careful about 'hidden' sugars, such as may be found in condiments and sauces.

PROOF

Just to prove how important the 'no-sugar' part of the diet is in dealing with Candida, consider the evidence from one trial in which 100 women with thrush and vaginitis were carefully studied. First, it was found that the higher the levels of glucose and lactose (milk sugar) intake, the worse their condition became, and when they were placed on a diet which eliminated simple sugars and dairy produce (because of the lactose) their condition improved dramatically. A separate research study showed that it was not possible to grow Candida albicans in human saliva until sugar was added.

It is, therefore, absolutely essential that in order to control Candida albicans you need to limit sugar in all forms – very strictly – for some months, and to pay attention to those things which boost blood sugar – such as caffeine, tobacco, alcohol and stress.

THE BLOOD-SUGAR ROLLER-COASTER

Some of the symptoms which are attributed to the presence of Candida overgrowth are often found to relate more directly to imbalances in blood-sugar levels, and it is important to understand this aspect of the way your body works.

The body needs to maintain a steady level of sugar in the blood to be available as an energy source for body activities, and this is best achieved by eating a balanced diet which allows for a slow and stable sugar release.

When simple sugars (refined sugar) are consumed there is a very rapid rise in blood sugar, and because it is dangerous to have a high level of sugar in the blood (a constantly high blood-sugar level is a diabetic state) the pancreas produces insulin to bring things down to safe levels. Sudden fluctuations – with swings up and down of blood-sugar levels – cause symptoms such as mood-swing, fatigue, weakness, irritability, nervousness, and 'brain-fog'. It is in this sort of state that children (and many adults) are often seen to be hyperactive and also hyper-irritable.

HOW WE HANDLE LOW BLOOD-SUGAR LEVELS

When blood-sugar levels have been pushed down by insulin, and all or any of these low blood-sugar symptoms start to appear, a 'quick-fix' is often sought to boost sugar again, either from an obviously sweet source (candy, cake, soft drink, etc.) or from a stimulant such as coffee, tea, cola, chocolate, alcohol or tobacco.

Another way of boosting sugar when it is low is to live or work in such a way as to encourage a feeling of being stressed, since this too causes adrenal stimulation and a sugar boost. This pattern of recurrent sugar boosts is one which is ideal for encouraging Candidiasis.

It is usually when blood-sugar is low that cravings are noticed, and the best way to eliminate these cravings (for sweets, chocolates, carbohydrate-rich foods, etc.) is to maintain a stable blood-sugar level by eating a diet which avoids simple refined sugars, by following a little-and-often policy of eating (five small meals daily instead of three big ones) and/or the use of substances which boost blood-sugar levels artificially.

SUGAR'S NEGATIVE EFFECT ON IMMUNE FUNCTION

One further negative effect of a sugar-rich diet is that the foods which provide this sort of 'empty-calorie' nutrition are usually deficient in the essential vitamins and minerals needed for normal functioning of the body. Nutritional imbalances of this sort have major effects on how we function, and especially on our defence systems. It has been shown that a high refined sugar intake severely weakens that aspect of the immune system which protects you from bacterial and viral infections. If you are prone to more colds and other infections than is usual, it may be that your sugar intake is compromising the ability of your defence mechanisms to operate efficiently.

If, as a part of the symptom picture which you display, you recognize that some of your symptoms relate to low blood-sugar (hypoglycaemia) you should consider taking professional advice as well as adopting the strategies suggested in this book. There are specific nutrient supplements (such as chromium) which can be taken for a short period to assist in restoring a more balanced blood-sugar picture.

WHAT SUBSTITUTES ARE THERE FOR SUGAR?

The best answer is to cultivate the opposite of a sweet-tooth, to learn to enjoy flavours other than sweet ones and to eventually come to find sweetness unpleasant.

Aspartame is a sweetener which does not encourage yeast activity. However, its regular use may carry as yet unidentified risks. There are many recorded cases of individuals using 'diet' drinks (sugar-free but using aspartame as a sweetener) developing severe headaches and mood swings, so any aspartame usage should be little and infrequent.

IS FOS AN ACCEPTABLE SWEETENER?

There is a newly identified amino-sugar product which does not 'feed' yeast, and which is actually shown to encourage the friendly bacteria in their recolonization. This is fructo-oligosaccharide (FOS) which is found in large amounts in fruit and vegetable fibre, and is particularly plentiful in Jerusalem artichokes. FOS tastes sweet, and can be added to food for this purpose in the safe knowledge that it will not aggravate Candida problems, and will actually encourage the friendly bacteria to perform their important roles more efficiently.

The recipes and menus in this book emphasize the need for a low sugar intake.

CHAPTER TWO

Yeast-free Diet – Yes or No?

The longer you have had a yeast overgrowth problem in the intestinal tract the more likely it becomes that your body will have become sensitized to yeast, and will react in an allergic manner to any food, drink or inhaled substance which contains yeasts or moulds.

Amongst the most obvious of these foods will be aged-cheese (blue cheese in particular) and wines. If you react to these – with symptoms such as increased fatigue, digestive disturbance (especially increased bloating), headaches, mood swings or an increase in yeast infection activity such as vaginitis or thrush in the mouth – then it is extremely likely that you have become sensitized to yeasts and moulds.

YEAST-BASED FOODS DO NOT ENCOURAGE CANDIDA

It is important to realize and understand clearly that avoiding foods which are derived from, or contain, yeast or which have a high likelihood of a mould presence (see below) is only necessary if you react adversely to such foods. Contrary to what is suggested by so many badly informed experts, yeast-based foods do not increase Candida activity.

In cases of adverse reaction their avoidance is recommended simply because they make you feel bad and put a strain on your immune system which is trying to get you better; not because they encourage Candida – which they do not.

Before looking at lists of foods and substances which contain yeast and moulds you need to appreciate how to identify allergy/intolerance/sensitivity reactions and how to handle foods which produce such reactions. This is achieved by means of 'elimination' and/or 'rotation' diets.

TRUE ALLERGIES

It is likely that you will already be aware of foods to which you are truly allergic, and to which you respond with symptoms such as asthma, hives, marked palpitations and immense fatigue. These are commonly foods which you do not eat too often, and to which you have a long-term sensitivity – seafood and peanuts are two of the commonest culprits. Medical tests are available which can identify the culprits in any particular case and, of course, once identified they should be carefully avoided.

MASKED ALLERGIES

Experts in allergy have come to realize that many people have allergies, intolerances or sensitivities to foods and substances which they consume daily or many times a day. Their reactions to these foods is usually muted – chronic, rather than acute as in the case of an obvious allergy.

A masked allergy may produce a wide range of symptoms – the most common of which are nasal irritation and congestion, allergic shadows under the eyes (dark rings), fatigue, digestive symptoms and/or pain, headache, joint and muscular pain and stiffness, irritation of the bladder, mood swings and a range of nervous system symptoms.

It is thought that when such symptoms are chronic, a masked allergy should be suspected. Because the substance/food is being reacted to many times a day, the degree of the reaction is less violent and takes the form of a low grade symptom which the individual assumes is 'just the way I'm made', and does not recognize it as an allergy.

A hopeful thought is that masked allergies can disappear if you become desensitized to the substance, but 'true' allergies are usually with you for life.

ELIMINATION AND ROTATION

Usually a masked allergy will not show up during normal medical allergy testing, which makes its unmasking a more difficult task. What is required is for the food or substance to be eliminated from the diet altogether for at least five days (it usually takes this long for all traces of a food to be removed from the system and digestive tract) before there is a challenge – in which the food is reintroduced to see what reaction occurs.

If the symptoms ease or vanish during the elimination phase of the test and recur when the challenge occurs, this is a reasonable proof of a masked allergy. The food should then be avoided for some months to allow desensitization to take place. Thereafter it can often be reintroduced in a rotation pattern (once in five days) without problems and may gradually be safely reincorporated into the normal diet.

COMMON ALLERGENS

Apart from yeast-based or yeast-containing foods, which should be avoided altogether for some months if you are sensitive to them, the commonest foods which are involved in masked allergy are wheat (and often all grains), dairy foods (milk in particular), citrus foods, eggs, corn, soy products, chicken, beef, sugar, chocolate, antibiotic medication and food additives and colouring.

A clue to where to begin in the detective work associated with unmasking these possible allergens may be found by asking yourself two questions:

'What foods do I eat most often, every day or several times a day?'

'What food(s) do I crave, or would I miss the most if it (they) was (were) removed from my diet?'

The answers to these questions will often give a direct pointer towards culprit foods which can then be tested by elimination, challenge and possibly rotation. It is beyond this book's purpose to advise in detail on the processes of elimination and rotation and you should consult a good book on this subject, or preferably a practitioner who deals with allergy, so that you can be advised as you work your way through the maze of identifying and unmasking allergen foods.

As for yeast elimination, this is very much a part of the focus of this book, and the following advice should be carefully considered by anyone who has a yeast/ Candida problem.

SHOULD YOU STOP ALL YEAST-BASED FOODS?

How much you are affected by yeast-related foods and substances depends on how long you have been affect- ed by Candida and how severely.

Many people whose symptoms improve when they markedly cut their sugar intake find that avoiding mushrooms, blue cheeses, yeast-based breads, alcohol and dried fruits (most dried fruit is covered in a layer of mould when seen under a microscope!) helps their symptoms even more.

It is worth experimenting by cutting out altogether those foods which have been identified as having yeasts in them or on them, and then – if benefits have been found – leaving them out for several months at least before a slow reintroduction of selected items is tried. If something is then tolerated without symptoms when you once again start eating it, it can be left in the diet in a rotation pattern (once in five days) at which time another food should be reintroduced.

Expert advice suggests that if you have had a Candida problem for some time, and if the symptoms include digestive irritation, you should drop from your diet all foods containing yeast or moulds, as listed at the end of this chapter, for the duration of your anti-Candida diet, a period of at least three months.

However, you could instead try testing a limited reduction of the most obvious of these foods, to see whether you feel better, or you could consult someone to help you identify whether an intolerance exists, before going through the complicated process of elimination as described above.

A sensitivity/intolerance can also be identified by means of a direct challenge in which on an empty stomach, having carefully avoided yeast of all sorts for five days, you consume a portion of the substance/food to be tested and then assess the return of symptoms and/or monitor your pulse rate (a big increase or marked drop in pulse rate occurs during an allergic reaction).

This sort of challenge should only be carried out under direct supervision from a qualified practitioner.

It is far safer for anyone who may be yeast intolerant/sensitive to eliminate as many culprits from the diet as possible and to keep off these for at least three months.

FOODS TO AVOID IF YOU ARE YEAST SENSITIVE

- All mushrooms and fungi (including truffles).
- All cheeses with the exception of natural cottage cheese (unless you are sensitive to dairy foods).
- All dried fruits (for their high mould content) as well as their high sugar content.
- Avoid all nuts (high in mould) *unless you open their shells yourself and they are current year's crop.* Avoid all nut butters for the same reason.
- Never eat peanuts (or peanut butter) whether you shell them yourself or they are already shelled – their mould count is both very high and highly toxic.
- All breads, pastries, cakes and biscuits containing yeast (look instead for soda bread, unleavened bread, sourdough bread, Ryvita, rice cakes, oat cakes, pumpernickel).
- All malted foods – drinks, cereals and sweets.
- Any left-over food not refrigerated.
- Pickled and smoked products (including corned beef, smoked salmon, sausages).
- Any sauces or condiments which have a yeast content (read the labels!).

- Tea and coffee (both stimulate sugar release and are high in mould presence).
- Food supplements based on yeast (read all labels, many B-vitamins in particular are yeast based).
- Fermented products such as vinegar, wine, beer, spirits, liqueurs and cider.

CHAPTER THREE

What Can You Eat?

If your anti-Candida diet eliminates sugary foods, and possibly all those foods associated with yeast and moulds (see previous chapter), you might well wonder what is left to eat.

The fact is that what is left, unless there are specific intolerances/sensitivities or allergies, is a highly nutritious and varied selection of foods.

An anti-Candida diet should include:

- Almost all vegetables.
- After the first few weeks of the diet, most fruits (exceptions during the whole of the diet are very sweet fruits such as melons and sweet grapes). Avocado pears can be eaten during all of the diet, with the other (not sweet) fruits being reintroduced after three weeks or so. Two to three pieces of fruit daily are suggested.
- Most proteins, including **fish**, **meat** and **poultry** – but avoid smoked and processed versions as well as any which are intensely farmed and therefore are

likely to contain antibiotic or steroid residues (as well, almost certainly, as antibiotic-resistant bacteria). This means seeking out free-range and organic sources of meat. Most supermarket chains carry at least some organic (free range) poultry and often some organic meat – especially following the BSE disaster.

- Although very little milk, because of its sugar (lactose) content, and milk products, especially cheese, because of its fungal connections, should be included in your diet, **live yogurt**, particularly if it derives from goats or sheep is an exception and is usually well tolerated and helpful. **Butter** is also usually well tolerated and, because it is low in milk sugars, it is not contraindicated on an anti-Candida diet. Substitutes for milk include **soya**, **rice** and **oat milk**, all of which are tasty and nutritious.

- Most **whole grains** (barley, oats, rye, wheat, millet, as well as rice and buckwheat) – take care though over the age and possible mould contamination of all such products. Avoid refined grains (white rice, flour, etc.) because they act much as sugar in boosting blood-sugar levels.

- All **pulses** (bean family), **nuts** (freshly shelled, unprocessed) and **seeds** with the exception of any which are mould contaminated. If you are moving towards a vegetarian diet, or following one, it is important to ensure that you eat a daily quantity of combinations of grains and pulses or nuts/seeds so that the full complement of protein-forming amino acids are present. Tofu (made from soya beans) is an excellent protein and can be combined with almost any other foods being cooked (stir fried, steamed, etc.) and will take on the flavour of that food.

- Condiments such as **sea salt** or very small amounts of black pepper. Most spices are heavily mould contaminated and should be used sparingly. Salad dressings are undesirable but you can safely use **pure olive oil** (or safflower, or sunflower or flaxseed oils) together with freshly squeezed **lemon juice**, for vegetable and salad dressing. Olive oil is actually antifungal, but use only cold-pressed, virgin oil.

WHAT CAN YOU DRINK?

Fruit juice needs to be restricted on an anti-Candida diet because it boosts blood-sugar levels, as do all drinks which contain caffeine (tea, coffee, chocolate, cola drinks). These are undesirable because they stimulate adrenal function and so increase sugar levels (see Chapter 1). Alcohol is also highly undesirable, and most herbal teas are mould contaminated. Most tap water is considered to be polluted with petrocarbons and heavy metals in all industrialized countries. Filtered or bottled water is therefore thought best by most experts on health enhancement.

Select from the following:

- Pure water (filtered or bottled).
- Organic bottled (or freshly homemade) vegetable juices are nutritious and delicious. Avoid large amounts of pure carrot or beetroot juice as these are sugar-rich (and therefore sweet). V–8 vegetable juices are relatively pure and nutritious.
- Diluted Aloe vera juice (this has antifungal properties and can be added to water – see below).
- Lemon water (using juice from freshly squeezed lemons).
- Antifungal teas (such as Taheebo – also known as Pau D'Arco, see below – and chamomile).
- 'Diet' soft drinks – not colas – **in small quantities** because they contain artificial sweetening agents such as saccharine or aspartame and not sugar. These are not recommended but are safe as far as the anti-Candida diet is concerned. Avoid these (or have very little) if they contain citric acid.

WHAT ABOUT FOOD COMBINING?

For many people with digestive and more complex health problems a solution, at least in part, is found by carefully selecting which foods to eat together, and which to eat separately.

Based on the work, over half a century ago, of Dr William Howard Hay, an American physician, this approach to nutrition is known variously as the 'Hay Diet' and 'Food Combining'.

While aspects of the theories which support food combining remain controversial, there is little doubt about its efficacy in many cases, and if you have digestive distress there may be an advantage in incorporating some aspects (or all) of the guidelines (see below) into your eating plan.

The broad principles which guide selection of foods in this system are as follows:

- Proteins (fish, poultry, meat, eggs, cheese, nuts, etc.) should be eaten alone or with green leafy vegetables.
- Most important: starchy foods (potato, corn, beetroot, carrot or grains – including bread) should never be eaten at the same time as proteins (fish, poultry, meat, eggs, cheese, nuts, etc.). An exception is a grain and nut mixture. Starchy foods combine well with green vegetables.
- Rice (whole, brown) can also be eaten with protein meals.
- Fruits should be eaten alone, not with any other type of food (proteins or carbohydrates) although they combine fairly well (but not perfectly) with vegetables.
- Nut, seed and pulse combinations (the vegan way of putting together all the amino acids to form protein) can be eaten with all vegetables.

The most important lesson from the study of food combining is the separation wherever possible of starches/carbohydrates and proteins.

Some additional basic rules include:

- Buy organic foods if at all possible, and vegetables and fruits (when they re-enter your diet after a month or so) should be completely peeled if they are not organic.
- Remember, though, that organic foods go off faster than chemically treated ones, so store well – refrigerate and use airtight containers.
- Try to prepare food just before eating it.
- Cook vegetables by steaming, lightly boiling, stir frying, baking or stewing, but not by frying or over-boiling.
- Since all yeast-based foods are off-limits for many people on an anti-Candida diet, seek out yeast-free versions. If you are wheat-sensitive, experiment with non-yeasted rye bread as an alternative.

BASIC RULES OF HEALTHY EATING

Before examining some important antifungal foods, and having looked briefly at what it is safe to eat, there is some value in considering how to eat. The following simple guidelines may individually seem obvious, but experience shows that for many of us many of them are just not observed.

- Eat slowly, and chew thoroughly.
- Try to have a few moments of quiet before meals, perhaps breathing slowly and deeply. Your digestive system will thank you for it.
- Avoid eating altogether if you are upset, angry, or

in a rush. You will be better off having a steady walk, or in some other way calming down and relaxing, rather than placing food into a digestive system which cannot digest – which is what happens under these circumstances.

- If possible, don't drink with your meals, and avoid very hot or very cold drinks (or foods).
- Ensure that you drink not less than two litres of pure (not tap) water daily, irrespective of whatever other liquids you are also consuming.
- Eat little and often ('grazing') if this pattern suits you better than set, large meals.
- Based on the combining rules listed above, try to eat obviously starchy foods and proteins at separate meals.
- For the same reasons avoid eating fruit with other foods (banana, papaya and avocado are exceptions – it is all right to eat banana with other starches (porridge for example), avocado with protein and papaya with almost anything – since it contains vast amounts of digestive enzymes and is well tolerated by most people in any combination).

SPECIAL ANTIFUNGAL FOODS

Reference has already been made to several foods having specific antifungal properties. The 'super foods' already mentioned include olive oil, Aloe vera juice and Taheebo tea, and to these can be added garlic, onions and chives. A brief note on each of these will help to emphasize their importance.

Although the attack on Candida requires that specific substances be used to kill the yeast, it is obviously highly desirable for the regular diet to contain foods and drinks which further this objective.

Aloe Vera Juice

The juice of this desert plant contains antifungal properties as well as having a soothing effect on the digestive tract. The pure juice needs to be kept refrigerated, and several teaspoons daily in water are recommended as part of an anti-Candida campaign.

Chamomile Tea

This soothing tea (it helps relaxation and sleep), made from the flowers of chamomile, is antifungal and highly recommended as a substitute for regular tea.

Garlic

Garlic extracts kill most fungal organisms, and the taking of capsules (two to four daily) of garlic (deodorized to avoid social problems) as well as the regular eating of as much raw garlic as can be tolerated (cooked garlic loses much of its efficacy) is suggested as a major feature of any anti-Candida programme. The evidence for its antifungal qualities is well documented. However, its benefit goes beyond this since it helps to lower blood pressure, remove excessive cholesterol and generally acts as a detoxifying agent. Many people report digestive upsets when they first increase their garlic intake. This often relates to the 'die-off' of yeast rather than any harmful side-effect of eating or taking it, and so should be ignored since it will usually subside in a few days.

Onions, leeks and chives have a similar if somewhat lesser effect on Candida, and should also be included in the diet.

Live Yogurt

The bacteria used to make yogurt (Thermophilus and Bulgaricus) are not normal residents of our intestinal tracts, but Bulgaricus in particular is known to assist our own friendly bacteria to thrive, so yogurt which still has live cultures in it is very useful (many forms are heated after the making to give a longer shelf life, thus killing the bacteria). Note that when commercial yogurt is marketed as 'containing acidophilus or bifidus' this means that a small amount of these important friendly bacteria have been added after the making of the product, since they cannot themselves produce the changes which are needed to turn milk into yogurt. Nevertheless, regular consumption of live yogurt is a helpful addition to an anti-Candida diet.

Olive Oil

Olive oil contains oleic acid which has antifungal properties. It also assists in preventing the yeast form of Candida from transforming to its aggressive mycelial form. Several tablespoons daily are recommended, on salads, in cooking or neat.

Taheebo (Pau D'Arco) Tea

This extract from a South American plant (Tabebuia avellanedae) has a long native tradition as an antifungal agent, and several cups daily are suggested in addition to the chamomile tea already mentioned.

CHAPTER FOUR

Anti-Candida Supplements & Herbs

The diet for controlling Candida is simple. It should ...

- ... contain as little sugar of all sorts as possible,
- ... be low in simple carbohydrates (refined flour, white rice, etc.),
- ... possibly contain no yeast-derived foods (remember, only if you are sensitive to these do they need to be removed from the diet),
- ... and avoid allergens (and foods which produce sensitivity reactions).

If these elements are in place it is then necessary to add the vital part of the overall assault – a strategy which will safely and effectively kill off the yeast and repopulate the digestive tract with high quality friendly bacteria (known as probiotics).

This part of the programme often requires expert guidance since each person's level of health and their ability to handle the process of yeast dying off (and the need to detoxify this) is likely to be a little different from anyone else's.

There may also be quite significant differences from one person to another in the amount of irritation which the invading yeast might have caused to the delicate lining of the intestinal wall. If this is severe it can make recolonization by acidophilus and bifidobacteria difficult, leading to the need for taking specialized substances and herbs to assist in healing the intestinal wall.

The suggestions that follow are therefore provided to indicate the type of substances and products which may need to be used in any given case and are not specifically prescribed for everyone.

An anti-Candida approach, an example of which is outlined below, should be followed quite strictly (together with the dietary pattern outlined in previous chapters) for not less than three months, and possibly longer, depending on the response.

In most instances, quantities to be taken are not given in the lists below because individual needs should always be considered. Where quantities have been given, these are the most commonly suggested levels of intake, and may be varied under special circumstances following expert advice.

ANTI-CANDIDA STRATEGY

Choose from the following as appropriate:

- Caprylic acid (this is an antifungal coconut plant extract).

- Grapefruit seed extract – especially if parasites are also present in the gut.
- High potency garlic capsules.
- Herbal extracts of echinacea, hydrastis and berberine.
- Extract of Artemesia absynthium (antifungal and anti-parasitic).
- Biotin – 500 micrograms twice daily.
- Pau D'Arco and/or chamomile tea – several cups of each daily.
- Aloe vera juice – two teaspoons twice daily in water.
- Olive oil – two tablespoons daily at least.

To Encourage Repopulation of Intestinal Flora

Use all of the following:
(See the special notes at the end of this chapter on probiotics)

- Between meals (three times daily) take a half teaspoon each of high quality, freeze dried, L. acidophilus and Bifidobacteria (powder or capsule form).
- Once a day take a half-teaspoon (or good quality capsule) of L. bulgaricus, the yogurt forming bacteria, as this encourages L.acidophilus and Bifidobacteria to colonize.
- One to two tablespoons daily of fructo-oligosaccharides (FOS) to encourage bacterial recolonization.

General Nutritional Support

- One soundly formulated, yeast-free, multivitamin/ multimineral supplement to provide at least the RDA (recommended daily amount) for all the major nutrients.
- One to two tablespoons daily of flaxseed oil as a source of essential fatty acids.

A wide range of other supplements are available to assist in recovery from Candidiasis. Expert advice is usually needed before selecting what is appropriate, so they should not be self-prescribed.

These include help in:

- Rebalancing glucose (sugar) tolerance (chromium polynicotinate) to help maintain stable blood-sugar levels (see Chapter 1).
- Encouraging better digestion (digestive enzymes, herbal products such as Swedish Bitters, peppermint oil).
- Improving liver function (specific amino acids such carnitine and taurine) as well as herbal products (Silymarin, dandelion and/or artichoke extracts).
- Detoxification (beetroot extracts, etc.).
- Healing inflamed gut lining (rice bran oil, N. acetylglucosamine, butyrates).
- Supporting regeneration of intestinal tissues (zinc, magnesium, vitamin C and vitamin A supplements).

COST?

If cost is an issue (few of the nutrients suggested above can be prescribed under new NHS regulations) then the absolute minimum which can successfully be used to control Candida, in combination with the dietary programme (no sugar, etc.), is as follows:

- One good antifungal (caprylic acid for example).
- Acidophilus and Bifidobacteria plus FOS (fructo-oligosaccharide) biotin or olive oil.
- A good multimineral/multivitamin.
- If the gut lining is inflamed – N. acetylglucosamine.

NOTES ON PROBIOTICS

As already mentioned, amongst the most important part of the anti-Candida diet is the need to restore a healthy flora to the intestinal tract. In normal health, you have living in your digestive tract approximately 1.5 kilos in weight of over 400 different species of bacteria, and it is true to say that our very lives depend upon the activities of these organisms, most of which provide us with useful services in return for the food and accommodation we provide them with.

The following is a summary of the tasks they perform, when they are in good health:

- They manufacture B-vitamins such as biotin, niacin (vitamin B_3), pyridoxine (B_6) and folic acid.
- They provide the enzyme lactase which digests milk-based foods.
- They help to predigest the protein in milk products in which they are consumed (yogurt, for example).
- They produce powerful anti-tumour products.
- They help to keep control of undesirable bacteria and yeasts which may try to colonize the digestive tract; which is why yeast can spread when the friendly bacteria have been damaged – by antibiotics, for example.
- They enhance bowel function.
- They improve immune function (especially in the very young).
- They are an excellent treatment for food poisoning.
- They detoxify ammonia and other toxins in the gut.
- They help to control cholesterol levels.
- They improve absorption of nutrients from the digestive tract.
- They act as a protective medium when we are exposed to radiation.
- They take part in oestrogen recycling in women, and so play a major part in reducing menopausal problems.
- They have been shown to be useful when supplemented in the treatment of allergies, psoriasis, rheumatic conditions, cancer, skin complaints, cystitis, colitis, irritable bowel syndrome – and, of course, thrush and Candidiasis.

CARE IS NEEDED IN SELECTING SUPPLEMENTAL PROBIOTICS

Many of the products being marketed as containing acidophilus and/or bifidus are less than desirable. Some are actually potentially harmful, especially when they contain cocktails of bacteria, and not just those which are essential.

The following are the things you should look for, or ask about, when buying these products:

- Are the organisms in the product normal residents of the digestive tract (L. acidophilus and Bifidobacteria, for example) or are they transients (L. bulgaricus, for example)? Know what you are buying and why.
- Can they survive the digestive process (are they microencapsulated?) or are they meant to be taken away from mealtimes to ensure safer passage?
- Are the strains you are buying known to be able to attach to the gut surface and colonize? If not, avoid them.
- Are there present in the bacterial product undesirable (or useless) organisms such as S. faecalis, S. faecium and L. casei? If so, avoid purchasing the product as these additional bacteria are usually included to bulk up the product, to give it longer shelf life, but not to help you or your health.
- Does the container in which they are purchased carry a guaranteed potency – a definite number of

colonizing organisms – usually expressed as so
many billions per gram?

- And does this guarantee apply up to a specified
  expiry date? If not, avoid the product.
- Is the container made of dark glass and not plastic
  (avoid plastic as it is porous and the freeze dried
  organisms will deteriorate)?
- Is refrigeration recommended for the product? If
  not, do not buy it.
- Is the product a powder or capsule? Avoid tablets,
  as the tablet-making process damages the bacteria.
- Was the product centrifuged when separating the
  bacteria from the 'soup' in which they were
  grown? If so, avoid them as this damages the
  delicate organisms.
- If you are dairy sensitive, ensure that the organisms
  were cultured on a non-dairy base (soya,
  carrot, etc.).

Probiotic products are not cheap, and many unscrupu-
lous manufacturers try to take advantage of the relative
ignorance which exists about just what is and what is
not desirable and necessary. I hope the information and
suggested questions listed above will help you to make
a better choice.

CHAPTER FIVE

The Anti-Candida Breakfast

Since the digestive tract is the main site of overgrowth of Candida albicans it is most important to ensure that it functions as well as it possibly can during the recovery stages. Your diet should be one which provides a reasonable level of fibre, adequate levels of essential nutrients and as little as possible of anything likely to encourage yeast activity. These requirements are fulfilled by the breakfast choices which follow.

It is important to eat slowly, to chew well, and to make sure that you eat three meals daily (unless there are low blood-sugar problems, in which case more frequent snack-type meals are appropriate).

If on some days you really don't feel like eating, then you shouldn't. Instead, have something such as a vegetable juice or a little live yogurt – and rest. If your loss of appetite continues, get advice.

For the first three to four weeks avoid choosing menus involving fruit. Also, for 'milk' use soya milk (unsweetened), rice milk – 'ricedream' (although this tastes on the sweet side) or oat milk. Many of the suggestions are straightforward and do not require recipes, but in some cases full recipes are given later in the chapter and this is indicated.

BREAKFAST CHOICES

If sweetening is required for any of the following, add fructo-oligosaccharide (FOS) – see the end of Chapter 1.

- Oatmeal porridge (made with water) – add cinnamon and/or freshly ground or whole cashew nuts or almonds (see recipe later in this chapter).
- Natural live yogurt (low fat) to which add one or two tablespoons of cold-pressed flaxseed oil, which should be blended well with it.
- Mixed seed and nut 'power' breakfast (see recipe later in this chapter).
- Toasted seed mixture with yogurt (see recipe later in this chapter).
- Wholewheat or rice or oat pancakes (see recipe later in this chapter).
- Two eggs – any style except fried or raw (raw egg white contains a substance which prevents Biotin from functioning normally (see Introduction).
- Wholewheat or millet or rice flakes (unsugared), or unsugared fresh home-made muesli mixture, and live yogurt. Take care not to use commercial muesli because of the likelihood (almost certainty) of the seeds and nuts being rancid and the dried fruit being mould contaminated (see recipe later in this chapter).

- Fruit, with particular emphasis on enzyme-rich examples such as avocado, papaya, mango, kiwi or pineapple from week 3 onwards (avocado is suitable from day 1 of the programme). All fruits, except very sweet ones such as melon and sweet grapes are acceptable after the first three weeks.
- Brown rice, moistened with olive or flaxseed oil, to which add fish (canned tuna or salmon, for example) or kedgeree – traditional Scots rice and fish dish (see recipe later in this chapter).
- Ryvita, rice cakes or yeastless bread or toast with humus or tzatzicki (see recipe later in this chapter).

RECIPES
Oatmeal Porridge and Nuts (optional)
(serves one)

Traditionally rolled oats, water and a touch of salt are all you need for this nourishing and satisfying start to the day. However, consider using cracked wheat, millet or rice flakes instead, for variety.

Ingredients:
1 cup oat (or rice or millet) flakes
2 cups water
Pinch of sea salt
(Optional – fresh or lightly roasted whole or grated
    almonds or cashews – to taste)
quarter teaspoon cinnamon

Method:

Place water and oat flakes in a saucepan, bring to the boil stirring constantly (prevents sticking to the pan). Once boiling, lower the heat, cover and allow to simmer for 20 to 30 minutes, stirring periodically.

Serve with cinnamon, plus whole or grated almonds or cashew nuts (fresh or lightly roasted).

Low-fat Yogurt and Flaxseed Oil

By blending flaxseed oil with the low-fat yogurt your digestion and absorption of the oil is enhanced. Full-fat yogurt will not as easily accept the additional oil, so be sure to seek out the low-fat varieties, and remember to choose live yogurt containing the friendly bacteria which will assist in recolonizing your digestive tract as Candida is being eliminated. This oil contains a high quantity of essential fatty acid and is very useful in health promotion in general and in recovery from a condition such as Candidiasis in particular.

Method:

To a standard size, individual serving (4 oz/115g) carton of yogurt add two tablespoons of cold pressed flaxseed oil and blend well by hand or machine.

Eat this on its own, or add several tablespoons of organic linseed (especially useful if constipation is a problem) or use as a dressing for cereal/seed mixture dishes shown below.

Mixed Seed and Nut 'Power' Breakfast
(serves one)

Variations on the theme of this recipe can be invented depending upon what ingredients are available – be creative!

Ingredients:
(choose three or more from the following)
1 tablespoon sunflower seeds
1 tablespoon pumpkin seeds
1 tablespoon linseed
½ tablespoon sesame seeds
½ tablespoon pine kernels
Contents of five almonds, walnuts or pecans
4 oz (115g) natural (ideally low-fat) yogurt
2 tablespoons cold-pressed flaxseed oil
(Optional – 2 tablespoons of either rice or millet or wheat flakes)

Method:
Soak the seeds overnight in a little water (just cover them). In the morning add the milled nuts and pine kernels and the flaked cereal (if desired). Add the yogurt and flaxseed oil mixture to make a very nourishing, energy-rich meal.

Toasted seed variation:
Place several tablespoons each of sunflower, flaked oats (or flaked millet or rice) and sesame seeds, as well as flaked almonds into a large roasting tin, onto which a little almond or sesame oil has been spread. Roast at

medium heat (170°C), turning the seeds periodically until they are golden brown. Use these whole or ground (coffee grinder) together with the yogurt/flaxseed oil mixture as an alternative, crunchy, breakfast.

If you roast larger quantities of this mixture than can be consumed at one meal, keep the balance in an air-tight glass container to prevent rancidity.

Pancakes (wheat, rice or oats)

Ingredients (for five pancakes):
1 cup wheat, oats or rice flakes
¼ teaspoon sea salt
1 teaspoon baking powder
1 egg
1½ tablespoons olive oil
1 cup rice, almond, oat or soya milk (use rice milk with rice pancakes, oat milk with oat pancakes)
½ cup water

Method:
Mix all the dry ingredients, and in a separate bowl beat the egg to which add the oil, plant milk of choice and water. Mix well.

Incorporate the dry ingredients into the liquid mixture and blend well together.

Lightly oil a frying pan and heat. When hot, pour batter into the pan and, when bubbles appear, turn the pancake. Cook till golden brown.

Serve with FOS or puréed, unsweetened apple, or stewed berries (cranberries, blue berries, etc.) once fruit is back in the diet after the first three to four weeks.

Muesli Mixture
(serves one)

Ingredients:

1 tablespoon each (organic if possible) oat, millet, rye,
   barley, rice and wheat flakes (assuming no sensitivity
   to these – choose from what is available and
   preferred)

½ tablespoon oat or wheat bran (if your digestive
   system accepts bran and especially if constipation is
   a problem)

½ tablespoon wheat or oat germ (the nutritious 'heart' of
   the grain)

2 tablespoons mixed seeds (sunflower, sesame, linseed,
   pumpkin, pine kernels) – fresh or roasted, whole or
   ground, as described in previous recipes

1 tablespoon flaked coconut

(After the first three weeks of the diet – fresh berries or
   stewed frozen cranberries, or mashed or sliced
   banana, or grated apple)

Appropriate milk substitute (rice, oats, soy)

(If desired – live low-fat yogurt)

Method:

Place the grain and seed selection into a bowl and soak
overnight covered (just) in filtered water. In the morning add the fruit and the wheat or oat germ and (if
desired) some oat or rice or soy milk or live low-fat
yogurt (with or without the flaxseed oil).

Kedgeree
(serves two)

Ingredients:
Cupful brown rice and two cups water
4 free-range eggs (hard boiled)
6 oz (170g) haddock, naturally smoked (not dyed),
    or salmon or cod

Method:
Cook the rice in twice its volume of water, and at the same time (in a separate saucepan) boil the eggs. Poach the fish for five minutes in a small amount of water in a separate pan which has been greased with olive oil. Once cooked, let the fish cool (the rice is still cooking) and then break it into flakes. Chop the peeled eggs into small pieces. When rice is ready, mix all the ingredients together and add a little black pepper to taste. Serve with stir-fried vegetables or on its own.

Humus (dip)
Humus is a middle-eastern dish made from chickpeas (which are particularly nutritious, iron rich and easily digested)

Ingredients:
4 oz (115g) chickpeas (dried)
2 tablespoons tahini paste (made from sesame seeds
    – obtainable from any health store and
    most supermarkets)
4 tablespoons olive oil
2 cloves garlic

Sea salt to taste
Lemon juice (one lemon)
Black olives (if desired)

Method:

Soak the chickpeas overnight, remove from water and add fresh water, bring to the boil and cook for 10 minutes before changing water again. Cook chickpeas until tender. The changing of the water eliminates the gas-forming enzymes which can make eating pulses a problem for many people, especially if they already have problems of bloating because of Candidiasis.

Place chickpeas into a bowl and add tahini, salt, garlic, lemon and 4 tablespoons warm water. Blend until creamy (using a food processor or pestle and mortar). If the consistency is too thick, add a little water to thin it. Place in serving bowl and refrigerate. Serve with black olives and use as a dip – with rice cakes, Ryvita or yeast-free bread or toast.

Tzatzicki (dip)

Ingredients:
8 oz (225g) low-fat live yogurt
2 cloves crushed garlic
Sea salt and black pepper to taste
2 tablespoons olive oil
1 teaspoon cider vinegar (optional)
half a cucumber, grated (skin and all)

Method:

Mix the crushed garlic with the salt and pepper and then add the oil (and vinegar if this is being used) in stages stirring gently until a blend is achieved. Add the grated cucumber, and chill before serving. Use as a dip (carrot or celery sticks or rice cakes or Ryvita or yeast-free bread or toast) on its own or at the same time as humus.

CHAPTER SIX

Candida Diet – Main Meals

Unless you have a wide range of food sensitivities/allergies/ intolerances, almost the entire vegetable kingdom as well as a wide range of protein sources are available for you to enjoy together with, after a few weeks, most fruits.

Before looking at main meal choices it is as well to re-emphasize the idea of seeking out organic sources of food. This is more than just an idealistic concept, and has immense implications for the anti-Candida programme.

Remember that most commercially produced eggs, and meat (and increasingly fish when it is farmed) contain residues of antibiotics and steroids – both of which encourage yeast activity by virtue of the damage they do to the friendly bacteria.

Remember also that, unless they are organic in origin, most fruit and vegetables (as well as grains) are loaded with chemical contaminants such as pesticides as well as having been treated to retard decay. These chemicals are harmful to the gut flora and therefore encourage Candida activity.

Look for organic fruit and vegetable sources and for really free-range eggs, poultry and meat, as well as for 'wild' fish sources. Even major supermarket chains now carry some of these, and as the negative effects of current farming practices become ever more evident, an inevitable increase in demand is sure to improve their availability.

MAIN MEAL CHOICES – VEGETARIAN OR NOT?

Keeping in mind the idea of 'food combining' (see Chapter 3), one of the two main meals of the day should be focused on a protein source and the other on a carbohydrate (starch) source, with appropriate vegetables, salads, etc. offering the accompaniment. Suggestions and recipes are given later in this chapter.

The speed with which you recover from a Candida problem will not be significantly influenced by your being vegetarian or not, as long as you follow the basic rules as outlined in previous chapters. Far more important than the type of your protein intake (bearing in mind what was said earlier about organic sources) are two key requirements which must be constantly emphasized.

• To avoid sugar-rich foods and those habits which encourage unstable blood-sugar levels, such as use of stimulants like tea, coffee, cola, chocolate, tobacco and alcohol.

- To follow the antifungal protocol outlined in Chapter 4.

WHAT'S AVAILABLE?

Clearly there can be problems associated with what is available when meal times come around. If you are obliged to eat in a canteen, or there are few local food outlets near your place of work, or there is very little time for a midday meal at all, you may have to consider taking a packed lunch.

Salads, home-made salad dressing (see recipe to follow), rice cakes, unyeasted bread or rolls, dips (see recipes for Humus and Tzatzicki in Chapter 5), fresh nuts, seeds, yogurt – are just some of the possible snack/lunch meals you can easily prepare at home and take with you to work. If facilities allow, home-made soup can be warmed at work as well.

If you are able to find suitable cafés and restaurants for a meal at midday (or evening) care is needed in what you choose. Avoid sauces and gravies, desserts, stuffing and anything you know to be likely to produce a sensitivity/allergy reaction.

BREAD?

For many people the most difficult part of an anti-Candida diet is avoiding yeast-based bread. Clearly, if you are sensitive to yeast, then bread made with it must be avoided for some time. Sourdough or soda breads do not have a yeast starter and are normally safe to eat for yeast-sensitive people.

It is also important that anyone who is wheat sensitive should avoid any bread containing wheat. Many rye breads, for example, are not pure rye but a mixture of rye and wheat. Check the content of what you are buying – pure rye or pure corn breads exist, but you have to find them.

Non-yeasted breads are now easily obtainable from health stores and many supermarkets.

LIGHTLY COOKED –
BETTER THAN RAW?

It is probably wise for anyone with a particularly sensitive digestive system to avoid raw salads for a few weeks at first and instead to focus on lightly steamed or stir-fried vegetables. Light cooking breaks down cellulose structures in the vegetables and allows easier access to the vital nutrients in them. Light does mean just that, a few minutes of stir-frying or steaming will not produce the softness (and sogginess) which is so much a feature of overcooked boiled vegetables – and this texture may come as a revelation to you. Ideally, vegetables should remain crunchy and firm with just the edge taken off their 'rawness'.

DRESSING FOR VEGETABLES AND SALADS

Commercial salad dressing should be avoided. Try some of the variations suggested in the recipe section later in this chapter.

ROTATE, BUT NOT OBSESSIVELY!

Remind yourself, by reading Chapter 2 again, of the importance of avoiding frequent repetition of any food during recovery from Candida overgrowth. Because the intestinal wall may have been irritated there exists the chance of absorption of proteins and other products of food as it passes through the tract – and of the development of sensitivities.

The more varied the diet the less likely this is to happen, and so a degree of rotation of foods is sensible. Rotation means that you try to space out the frequency with which you eat particular foods or families of foods. If possible you should try to choose different fruits, or sources of protein (meats for example) or grains so that a different one is eaten each day for five days, at which time the first can be eaten again.

Rotation patterns are ideal if no sensitivity already exists – although even if they do and especially if they are not too severe, rotation can be a way of incorporating 'problem' foods into the diet.

Examples

(It is assumed that all sources are free-range and/or organic)

	Grains	Proteins	Fruit	Vegetables
Monday	wheat	chicken	apples	peas/beans, etc.
Tuesday	millet	lamb	citrus	courgettes/squash
Wednesday	oats	fish	papaya	potatoes
Thursday	barley	eggs	berries	carrots
Friday	rye	seafood	banana	cabbage, etc.

On Saturday you can go back to wheat/chicken/apple/peas and beans, etc., so starting the rotation schedule again. A similar rotation schedule can be constructed for other food types (nuts, seeds, oils and so on).

Remember also that the examples given above are just that – examples – and that the list above is not a prescribed sequence which has some particular importance. In other words, the suggestions for Monday could just as appropriately have been wheat, lamb, papaya and carrots. Make your own lists based on the foods you like and those that are 'safe' for you.

If you are prone to sensitivity/intolerance reactions, then use of rotation patterns of eating can prove to be a useful exercise. Do not, however, become so obsessive over its application that it dominates your life. It is just one possible strategy (along with 'food combining') which can make reactions less frequent and less severe as you recover from the effects of Candida overgrowth.

The list of possible meals which follows is not meant to be comprehensive, but it offers thoughts and suggestions from which you can create an almost infinite variety of choices to suit your personal tastes and situation.

'SAFE' FOODS

Some people seem to be sensitive to almost everything. However, some foods have an almost universally 'safe' track record, in that few people find them a problem.

The famous 'lamb and pear' diet has been used for many years to begin the desensitization of people with multiple allergies, since few people react to either of these two foods, or to rice or buckwheat. Neither rice nor buckwheat are grains and they are usually well tolerated (if organic and whole – not polished). Many 'allergies' to wheat and vegetables in fact represent a sensitivity to the chemicals on and in them rather than the foods themselves.

Amongst fruits, the safest (apart from pears) seem to be tropical, enzyme-rich fruits such as papaya, mango, kiwi, pineapple and guava.

MAIN MEAL CHOICES

Many of the suggestions are simple to prepare and do not require recipes, but for those that do a detailed recipe is given later in the chapter. Wherever possible the principles of 'food combining' are adhered to in these suggestions, although this is not always the case.

- Home-made soup (see recipes later in this chapter).
- Mixed salad and/or vegetables and/or rice (or toasted rice cakes) or yeastless bread or toast (see recipes for salads and for cooked vegetable mixtures later in this chapter).
- Fish and green salad and/or cooked vegetables and/or rice (see recipe for savoury rice later in this chapter).
- Poultry or meat and green salad and/or cooked vegetables and/or rice.
- Vegetarian savoury, possibly including tofu (see recipes later in this chapter) and green salad and/or vegetables (regular cooking or stir-fried) and/or rice.
- Vegetarian stew (vegetables and tofu).
- Eggs and green salad and/or vegetables and/or rice.
- Dips (see recipes later in this chapter) with rice cakes or yeastless bread/toast or salad sticks (celery, carrot, cucumber, radish, etc.).
- Rice or millet or (if you are not wheat sensitive) regular wholewheat pasta (spaghetti, etc.) and home-made tomato-based sauce (see recipe later in this chapter).
- Safe desserts (see recipes later in this chapter).

SOUPS

There are a wide variety of canned, frozen and pack-aged, available for convenience. However, these are not suggested for use in an anti-Candida diet. The problem with most commercial soups lies in their host of additives, flavourings, colourings and preservatives, many of which are yeast-based or have the potential to produce negative effects on anyone with food intolerances. Home-made soups are easy to prepare and can easily be offered as a main meal in themselves. A few examples are provided below. Consult wholefood cookbooks for variations on these.

Remember some basic tips for soup making:

- Vegetarian soups can be made more nourishing by incorporating as a stock the water in which vegetables have previously been cooked.
- If meat or fish stock is being made, try to ensure that the bones being used to make this derived from organically reared of animals.
- There are some commercially produced yeast-free soup stocks – but you will have to search for these cubes or powders in health stores and/or specialist suppliers. Read labels carefully to ensure that the ingredients are safe for you.
- For soups which have a creamy texture add a little sheep's or goat's yogurt to the soup after the cooking is complete, ensuring that the liquid is no longer boiling so that curdling does not occur.
- Alternatively you could incorporate sheep's, goat's, soya or oat milk into the preparation early on.
- If you are using beans, especially red kidney beans, in any of the soup recipes, follow a rule of soaking these overnight, discarding the water, adding fresh

water and then part boiling them before again discarding the water just before adding them to the soup for the final cooking process. This complicated process eliminates gas-forming enzymes which have given beans a reputation which is all too familiar to people with digestive and bloating problems.

RECIPES
Potato Soup
(serves two to three as a main course)

Ingredients:
2½ lb (1.25kg) potatoes, peeled and diced
1 large onion, chopped
1½ pt (850ml) water
13 fl oz (370ml) sheep's, goat's or soya or oat milk
Sea salt and black ground pepper to taste
1 tablespoon natural yogurt

Method:
Place the potatoes and onion in a saucepan and cover with water. Simmer on a medium heat until the potatoes are tender, at which time cream these in a blender and then return the potatoes to the saucepan. Once again bring to the boil and add the milk and seasoning. Allow to simmer while stirring periodically until the soup is thick and creamy. Just before serving, add the yogurt to the bowl of soup. Serve with yeast-free toast, or Ryvita or rice cakes.

Chickpea Soup
(serves three as a main meal)

Ingredients:
1 lb (450g) dried chickpeas
2 tablespoons fresh or dried rosemary
Sea salt and ground black pepper to taste
7 fl oz (200ml) olive oil
Juice of one lemon or tablespoon natural yogurt

Method:
Soak the chickpeas for 24 hours, during which time change the water at least twice. Place in saucepan and cover completely with fresh water. Bring this to the boil and simmer for 30 minutes before changing to fresh, hot water. Resume cooking and change the water again 20 minutes later. Add the rosemary, salt, pepper and oil and allow to simmer until the chickpeas are very soft. Add lemon juice or yogurt just before serving.

Jane McWhirter's Quick-fix Soups
(quantities are per person)

Jane McWhirter has written an excellent book on Candida (*The Practical Guide to Candida*, All Hallows Foundation, 1995) which also gives names of practitioners throughout the UK treating the condition holistically. In this she gives a recipe for a rapidly prepared soup (20 minutes or so on average) which is in contrast to the fairly laborious (if delicious) chickpea soup described above. Obviously, this is an ideal approach for anyone who, because of their work or circumstances, cannot spend much time in preparation and cooking. I have slightly modified Jane's recipe in the outline given below.

Ingredients for soup base:
2 tablespoons olive oil (described by Jane as a 'slug')
Half an onion, diced
Clove of garlic, diced
Sea salt and ground back pepper to taste

Other ingredients:
Choose from those listed below or almost any other vegetable mixture. Quantities are rough estimates per person. Note that if the bean options are used, pre-preparation of these is essential to avoid gas. Soak overnight (at least) and pre-cook as in chickpea soup recipe above.

1 large or 2 small courgettes and 4 oz (115g) spinach, or
2 celery stalks, 2 oz (60g) cashew nuts and 1 (cored and peeled) cooking apple
6 oz (170g) freshly picked, young, tender nettles, or
1 large leek and 1 lettuce, or
Pulse soup (note – chop or shred all vegetable ingredients before cooking):
4 oz (115g) lentils, 2 oz (60g) ginger, tablespoon parsley,1 carrot, or
4 oz (115g) flageolet beans, 2 tomatoes, tablespoon basil, or
4 oz (115g) chickpeas, teaspoon cumin, 2 medium carrots, or
4 oz (115g) aduki beans, 2 medium-sized leeks, or

4 oz (115g) green lima beans, 1 large courgette, 3
  sprigs watercress

Method:
Stir-fry the onion and garlic in the olive oil for two minutes, or a little longer if you want a 'brown' soup (for
example the aduki bean option).

  Together with stock liquid (see notes above), or
water and seasoning, place the chosen ingredients (the
stir-fried onion and garlic as well as the choice of vegetables or pulses) into a saucepan and simmer until just
tender. Avoid excess stock/water, use just enough to
allow the ingredients to simmer without burning.
Remove from heat, and *when not very hot* blend in liquidizer (or put through a food processor by placing
solids in the machine having separated them from the
liquid, which you add back after processing is complete). If no processor or liquidizer is available, prepare
ingredients by finely chopping these before cooking.

  To the finished soup add a tablespoon of yogurt or
add a few tablespoons of cooked rice (especially to pulse
soups for complete protein source) or small pieces of
precooked rice-based or wheat or millet pasta.

SALADS

Salads offer quick, inexpensive (relatively) and potentially delicious and nutritious meal options. Unless your
digestive system really finds raw food difficult to cope
with, one salad meal a day is suggested. However, if you

cannot at this stage easily digest raw foods, use instead lightly cooked vegetables (see below) as a source of vital mineral and vitamin nutrients.

Dressings for Salad

Rather than using commercially prepared dressings, the following alternatives exist for putting zest into salads.

- Olive oil and juice of one freshly squeezed lemon or lime (2 parts oil to 1 part juice).
- Olive oil and juice of one freshly squeezed lemon or lime (2 parts oil to 1 part juice) plus one or two tablespoons of live yogurt.
- Olive oil and juice of one freshly squeezed lemon or lime together with a clove of crushed garlic and/or a little freshly ground black pepper.
- A variety of herbs can also be used , if they are fresh, to subtly alter the taste of the dressing – such as rosemary, thyme, oregano and basil, by placing a pinch of any of these into the mixture just before use.
- Tofu dressing can replace creamy mayonnaise-type dressings. You will need to blend the following ingredients into a creamy texture, by hand with a fork or using a blender – 4 oz (115g) tofu, the juice of a lemon, and black pepper to taste.

If you want to take a salad to work, find a small glass screw-top container for the ingredients for one of the oil based mixtures above. Shake before using on your salad lunch.

Ingredients for Salads

The list is almost endless, and you are urged to try to seek out tasty varieties of edible raw vegetables so that salads do not become boring. Major supermarket chains now sell ready-washed salad mixtures (more expensive but much more convenient than preparing them yourself) which contain, for example, a range of exotic leaf and other vegetables offering varieties of colour, texture and taste.

When preparing a salad try to vary:

COLOURS
- Beetroot, tomato or radish red
- Carrot orange
- Multiple types/shades of green
- Purple endive
- White cauliflower, chicory
- Rainbow options from different versions of pepper

TEXTURES
- Crunchy
- Chewy
- Soft
- Crisp

FLAVOURS
- Sweet as in carrot, tomato, grated raw beetroot, some onion varieties and sweet peppers
- Bitter as in chicory or dandelion
- Sharp as in watercress and rocket

- Nutty as in courgettes
- Smoky or sulphury as in cauliflower and kale
- Mustardy as in young nasturtium leaves or mustard and cress
- Tangy as in endive and celery
- Aromatic as in fennel, parsley, basil or mint
- Tart as in spring garlic or onion

SIZE AND SHAPE
- Grated carrot, beetroot or turnips
- Shredded leaves of endive, lettuce, cabbage and rocket
- Chunks such as sliced celery, fennel and apple
- Orbs such as radishes and small tender Brussels sprouts
- Circles such as onion or red, yellow and green peppers
- Spikes such as spring onions and spring garlic
- Tender sprouts such as alfalfa, mustard and cress, bean shoots
- Whole leaves of chicory, water cress, parsley

If you cannot create exciting salads out of a selection of these ingredients, settle for the prepacked, prewashed varieties sold by major supermarkets.

Remember the 'food combining' rules which suggest that for a sensitive digestion a salad (or cooked vegetables) will be better digested if eaten with either a protein (tuna, hardboiled egg, etc.) or a carbohydrate (jacket potato, rice cakes, savoury rice, etc.) *but not with both a carbohydrate and a protein.*

COOKED VEGETABLES AND VEGETABLE MIXTURES

The choices for cooking vegetables safely (i.e. retaining most of their nutritional value) are stir-frying, steaming and boiling.

Stir-fried food is excellent since the amount of time the food is heated is minimal (2 to 3 minutes is enough for most vegetables if chopped finely enough) which means that little of the value is lost. All you need is a wok (a deep frying pan will do) into which place a very little olive oil and heat until it is hot, at which time add the vegetables, stirring frequently with a wooden implement. By adding flavoursome ingredients such as garlic, ginger, onions, leeks and fennel, and also adding tofu (dice sized chunks of the soy based 'cheese' are suggested) a complete meal can be ready in under 10 minutes.

The advantage of steaming vegetables is that the retained food value is greater than when they are boiled. Steaming is also a quicker process than boiling, especially if you have a stainless steel steamer rather than using a sieve or colander placed over boiling water in a saucepan.

There are some simple rules to follow in either boiling or steaming vegetables:

- Place any root vegetables into the steamer (sieve, etc.), or the water itself if you are boiling, from the start, well before the water is boiling.

- On the other hand do not place any green vegetables in the steamer (or water) until the water is boiling.
- When steaming vegetables use a cover for most of the time, this retains the heat of the steam and speeds the process, and remember that the less time the vegetables are being heated the more nutrients they retain.
- If you decide to steam or boil the vegetables rather than stir frying them, cook them until they reach the degree of tenderness you prefer, drain and place on a serving dish.
- You can serve them directly or, alternatively, you can do so the Mediterranean way which means leaving them (covered) until they reach room temperature at which time dress with olive oil and lemon juice and serve. The advantage of this method is that vegetables can be conveniently prepared many hours before the meal. They also taste much better served at room temperature, compared with being served hot.

RECIPES
Stir-fried Vegetables
(serves one)

Ingredients:
1 diced green or red pepper
2 cloves garlic, sliced finely or crushed
ginger root (about 1 inch/2.5cm long), sliced or grated
1 carrot, sliced

1 small onion, cut lengthwise into eighths
1 courgette, sliced or diced
4 oz (115g) florets of broccoli or cauliflower
1 stalk of celery, sliced
2 teaspoons sesame seeds (optional)
3 oz (85g) diced tofu
Sea salt to taste
2 tablespoons olive oil

Method:
Place the oil and the ginger in the wok (or frying pan) and heat. When smoking slightly, add all other ingredients except the tofu, the seeds and the salt. Cook (stir frequently) for three minutes, then add the tofu and the sea salt for one more minute of cooking. Remove from heat and serve with a sprinkling of sesame seeds.

Greek Steamed Vegetable Salad
(serves one)

Ingredients:
(see alternatives following description of method)
1 carrot, well-washed and sliced
4 oz (115g) French beans, trimmed
Half fennel bulb, washed and cut into large pieces
1 globe artichoke, debearded, outer leaves removed
    and cut into eight small pieces
4 oz (115g) peas
1 medium-sized potato cut into six pieces
1 celery stick, strings removed and sliced
1 small beetroot, undercooked and diced
10 black olives

1 small Spanish onion
Olive oil, cider vinegar or lemon juice, sea salt and
   oregano for dressing

Method:
Place the carrot, beans, fennel, artichoke, peas and
potato into a steamer (a large sieve or a colander placed
over a saucepan of boiling water will do instead).

Steam for 10 minutes before adding the celery, and
allow to steam for a further 10 minutes. Place cooked
vegetables on serving dish and add the diced beetroot,
olives and raw onion, as well as the dressing which
comprises two to three tablespoons olive oil, one tablespoon cider vinegar (optional) or lemon juice, plus a
sprinkling of oregano and salt to taste.

Save the water in which you steam or boil and use
this for a soup stock or wait until it cools and drink it –
for the mineral content.

Alternative ingredients for this dish can include:
- Courgettes (sliced thickly if large or whole if small)
- Chicory (cut in half lengthwise)
- Spinach (whole or shredded)
- Turnip greens, beetroot tops, courgette tops and/or
  dandelion greens
- Cauliflower florets and/or Brussels sprouts (halved),
  etc.

Serve this 'cooked' salad on its own, with a protein
(tofu, fish, poultry, etc.) or with a carbohydrate (rye
toast, rice cakes, jacket potato, etc.).

Rice
(serves two)

There are many ways of preparing rice, and this book is not designed to offer comprehensive instruction. The method described below works adequately for brown (unpolished) whole grain rice.

Ingredients:
8 oz (225g) brown rice
2 pt (just over a litre) water
¼ teaspoon sea salt

Method:
Rinse rice in tepid water and place in saucepan covered by approximately 1.5 in. (4cm) of water, plus salt. Heat and bring the water to the boil. Once the water is boiling, reduce heat so that a gentle simmering is taking place. Don't stir the rice when cooking or it will become sticky. During cooking more water may be added if needed (different types of rice require more or less water) by pouring already boiling water onto the cooking rice. Approximately 45 minutes will be needed to produce fluffy cooked rice.

Savoury Rice Variation
(serves two)

After the cooking process various additions can be made to the rice, such as:

Olive oil (4 fl oz/115ml)
1 ripe tomato, chopped
1 onion, finely diced

1 clove of garlic, crushed
½ green pepper, diced
1 carrot, finely diced
¼ cup dry roasted sesame seeds

Method:
Cook the rice in the way described above. When the rice has been simmering for 30 minutes sprinkle the sesame seeds into the rice. The seeds should previously have been dry-roasted in an oven until they turn light brown.

At this time the diced and chopped tomato, onion and garlic should be sautéed or stir-fried for three minutes before the pepper and carrot are added for a further three minutes (use minimal oil to coat the pan or wok).

Once the rice is cooked, the vegetables should be gently added and mixed.

The savoury rice can be served hot, together with a meat, fish, poultry or vegetarian dish, or at room temperature with a salad.

SAVOURY MEALS (VEGETARIAN AND NON-VEGETARIAN)

A few examples are given below of the sort of main course someone with a Candida problem might enjoy.

• Vegetarianism is not in any way an obligation, although the variety of choices available to anyone

inclined towards a balanced vegetarian diet
is enormous.

- If meat, poultry, fish, seafood or eggs present no
digestive or intolerance/sensitivity or allergy
problems then these may be eaten regularly.
- In any case consider applying the rotation
suggestions outlined earlier in this chapter so that
the same food type is not eaten too frequently.
- One meal daily should include a good source of
protein from whatever derivation. This could
accompany the salad meal or be a cooked mainly
protein meal, in which case, if digestive problems
exist care is needed regarding what accompanies
the protein (no potatoes or bread or other strong
carbohydrate ingredients).
- If meat, poultry or fish is eaten, avoid factory-
farmed varieties (even factory-farmed fish – and
this means most salmon and trout – may have, as
does factory-farmed meat and poultry, undesirable
antibiotic and steroid contamination).
- Try to obtain 'organic' meat/fish/poultry/eggs –
free-range if possible and free of chemical
contamination.
- When cooking animal proteins, avoid fat as far as
possible and avoid frying (grilling, baking and
boiling are best).
- If vegetarian options are chosen, remember that to
provide the body with the full complement of
amino acids (the building blocks of protein) it is
necessary to combine pulses (bean family) with
grains (wheat, barley, oats, rye, millet) or seeds

(rice, sunflower seeds, pumpkin seeds, sesame seeds, nuts, etc.). A lentil dish, together with rice, would offer just such a mixture (rice 'goes' with most foods).

To summarize (whether vegetarian or not):

- Keep proteins away from obvious carbohydrates as best you can.
- Obtain chemical-free foods.
- Have one good protein meal each day (at least).
- Keep ringing the changes – varying the type of fish, meat, poultry so that you avoid intolerances.
- If these already exist, strictly avoid the culprit foods.

Examples of several *vegetarian savoury* dishes are given below. (It is assumed that everyone knows how to cook meat, poultry and fish so recipes for these have not been included.)

Roasted Butter Bean
(serves four – this freezes well so can be kept)

Ingredients:
1 lb (455g) butter beans
4 fl oz (115ml) olive oil
½ oz (15g) parsley, chopped
1 lb (455 g) canned tomatoes
6 cloves garlic, halved lengthwise
2 sticks celery, including leaves if possible, chopped

1½ onions, chopped
2 carrots, chopped
1 teaspoon paprika
Sea salt and black pepper to taste

Method:

Soak the butter beans overnight and then, after again washing them well, place in boiling water and cook for 30 minutes. At this time change the water and continue to cook for a further 30 minutes in the new water.

Place the cooked beans in an oven container which is at least 2.5 inches (6.5cm) deep, together with all the other ingredients. Mix well and cover with water. Cover the container with foil and place in an oven at 350°F/180°C (Gas mark 4) for one hour, after which time remove the foil and allow the beans to continue to cook until all water has evaporated and the beans are tender, with some browning and crispness to those on the top. Depending upon the relative hardness of the water and the quality of the beans the cooking time will vary.

Serve with a salad or savoury rice.

Lentil and Nut Loaf
(serves six, freezes well)

Ingredients:

8 oz (225g) lentils
1 large onion, chopped
8 whole garlic cloves
3 tablespoons olive oil
5 oz (140g) ground walnuts or almond and/or pine kernels

6 oz (170g) fresh bread crumbs (use cooked rice or
    millet instead if desired)
2 tablespoons tomato purée
1½ teaspoons oregano
3 tablespoons parsley, chopped
2 eggs
Sea salt and freshly ground black pepper to taste
Tomato, onion and parsley to garnish

Method:
Soak the lentils for several hours, rinse and place in a
saucepan and cover with cold water. Simmer gently for
20 minutes, by which time they should be tender. Drain
off surplus liquid. Separately fry the onion and garlic in
olive oil until lightly brown. Remove from heat and add
nuts, lentils, bread crumbs (or cooked rice or millet),
tomato pure, oregano, parsley, eggs. Mix well and season to taste with salt and black pepper.

Place a strip of foil on the bottom and on the sides of
a loaf tin, grease this with oil and place the mixture in
the tin. Cover the mixture with a piece of greased foil.

Bake in an oven at 350°F/180°C (Gas mark 4) for
one hour. After removing from the oven, leave the loaf
in the tin for a few minutes. Run a knife around the
edges and turn out the loaf. Garnish with tomato, onion
and parsley. Serve in thick slices with salad or cooked
vegetables.

DIPS

See recipes for Tzatzicki and Humus in the previous chapter. The two additional dip recipes which are provided below offer a choice which can be used for snack meals or main meals when eaten with salad (carrot and celery sticks) or rice cakes, for example.

Aubergine Dip

Ingredients:
2 large aubergines
13 fl oz (370ml) olive oil
8 fl oz (225ml) goat's, or oat or rice or soya milk
Lemon juice to taste
2 oz (60g) low-fat cottage cheese (optional)
Sea salt and freshly ground black pepper to taste
Tomato, black olives and parsley to garnish

Method:
Wash and dry aubergines and place in oven at 350°F/180°C (Gas mark 4) for 1 to 1½ hours. When cooked, remove and discard skin. Place the flesh in a mixing bowl and reduce to a creamy mixture using a fork. Then, using a pestle and mortar, add alternately the oil, milk (or substitute) and a little lemon juice. As these are added, work the ingredients well together. When the mixture is frothy, add the cottage cheese. Season with salt and pepper and place in a bowl which can be decorated with tomato, parsley and black olives.

Olive Dip

Ingredients:
1 lb (455g) black olives
3 fl oz (85ml) olive oil
6 cloves of garlic, crushed
2½ fl oz (70ml) lemon juice
1 tablespoon oregano
Black pepper
Lemon slices to garnish

Method:
De-pip the olives and place in blender/processor. Blend until they reach a creamy consistency. Add all other ingredients and mix well. Place in bowl and garnish with lemon slices.

SAUCES

Sauces are invaluable for lifting something which may be nutritious but tasteless, and yet they present particular problems for people with digestive disturbances in general and active Candidiasis in particular.

The sauce described below can be used on rice, on pasta (wheat if this is tolerated; if not a variety of soy, millet and rice pastas are now available in health food stores).

Home-made Tomato Sauce
(for use on rice, pasta, etc.)

Ingredients:
3 lb (1.4kg) canned tomatoes, including juice
1 oz (30g) parsley, chopped
1 teaspoon basil or three bay leaves
1 tablespoon FOS (see Chapter 1)
10 fl oz (285ml) olive oil
1½ large onions, chopped
2 oz (55g) garlic, chopped not crushed
Sea salt to taste

Method:
Place all ingredients into a non-stick saucepan, over medium heat, so that the contents simmer but do not boil. Simmer for between 1½ and 2 hours, stirring periodically, until all liquid has evaporated. The result will be a thick tomato sauce. This freezes well, so large quantities can be made at one cooking session.

DESSERTS

Sweet things taste nice, but most sweets are sugar-rich and therefore out of the question for the anti-Candida programme. So what's the solution?

We can use FOS for additional sweetness. However, at best, this should be a sometime thing since it encourages you to retain the desire for sweetness, and in the long run, even when Candida is once again controlled, it is not going to be a good idea to indulge in regular consumption of sweet things. So the two desserts suggested below are not necessarily sweet. Try them and hopefully adopt them.

One of the recipes below is derived from Jane McWhirter's book which was mentioned earlier (*The Practical Guide to Candida*). In it she credits Candida sufferer Sue Elliot with developing many recipes which she has described in her own book *Coping with Candida*. I am giving one of these below (the Pancake recipe) slightly modified.

The other recipe is from my wife's book *Greek Vegetarian Cooking*, and is for quince, baked in the oven, served with yogurt and nuts. This can clearly be modified to use cooking apples or pears instead, since availability of quince is limited to the late autumn and to specialist stores (Arab, Greek, etc.). Much less cooking time would be needed for apples, so experiment and keep an eye on the oven.

Dessert Pancakes

Ingredients:
4 oz (115g) 'safe' flour (rye, rice, barley, etc.)
2 eggs, beaten
2 tablespoons olive oil
7 fl oz (200ml) soya or oat milk

Topping:
Juice of 3 lemons and 3 tablespoons grated coconut
or Unsweetened cranberries (available frozen at better supermarkets)

or Grated fresh ginger (two teaspoons – or to taste –
   per serving)
or Cinnamon (quarter teaspoon per serving)
or Apple or pear purée, made without sweetening, or
   with FOS to taste

Method:
Sift the flour into a bowl and make a depression in the
centre of this, into which gradually beat in the other
ingredients (or liquidize all ingredients instantly).
When the batter is smooth, allow it to stand for half an
hour. Heat a small frying pan which has been lightly
oiled. Drop approximately 2 tablespoons of batter into
the pan and agitate this to form the desired shape.
Allow to cook until bubbles appear. The underside
should be golden brown by this time. Toss/turn the
pancake and cook the other side.

   Serve with one of the toppings listed above.
The method for the lemon and coconut option requires
that you blend together the lemon juice and desiccated
coconut, until smooth, and add to the pancakes.

Quince with Yoghurt and Nuts
(serves one)

Ingredients:
1 medium to large quince (or cooking apple?)
1 tablespoon freshly shelled walnuts
1 to 2 tablespoons thick, natural, ideally live, yogurt

Method:

Wash the fruit well and place in a preheated oven (300°F/150°C Gas mark 2) for 45 minutes. Remove from oven and open, discarding seeds and core. Serve together with nuts and yogurt while still hot. A little FOS (see Chapter 1) may be used if the sharpness of the taste (slightly sour) needs more camouflage. The yogurt and nuts should adequately soften this, though.

Index

abdominal bloating 3
acidophilus *see*
  Lactobacillus acidophilus
additives 57
alcohol 23
  and sugar reduction 7, 8,
    9, 10, 50
  and yeast-based product
    reduction 17, 20
allergen foods 16–20
allergies 14–20
Aloe vera juice 24, 27, 28,
  33
antibiotics 2, 3, 49, 71
antifungal foods 27–30, 50
appetite, loss 39
Artemisia absynthium 33
aspartame 11–12
avocado pears 21, 27, 41

bacteria, friendly 1–2
bananas 27

beans, dried, cooking 57–8
berberine (berberis) 33
Bifidobacteria bifidum
  (bifidus) 1, 6, 29, 32,
    33, 37
Biotin 2, 33
bloating 3
blood sugar:
  imbalances 9, 34, 50
  low 10, 11
bowel *see* gut
bread, yeast-based 17, 19,
  26, 51–2
breakfasts 39–48
buckwheat 55
bulgaricus see Lactobacillus
  bulgaricus
butter 22

caffeine 9, 23
caprylic acid 32

carbohydrates:
  in food combining 25,
    27, 50, 71, 72
refined 7–8
chamomile tea 28, 33
cheese 13, 17, 19
chemical contaminants 49,
    72
chewing 26, 39
chives 27, 29
chocolate 7, 10, 50
chronic fatigue 3
chronic muscle pain 3
coffee 7, 10, 20, 50
cola 24, 50
condiments 8, 19
constipation 3, 42
contraceptive pill 2, 3
cooking process 26, 52,
    65–6, 71
cost issues 35
Crook, Dr William 4

dairy produce 8
date sugar 8
desserts 77–80
detoxification 34
diarrhoea 3
'diet' soft drinks 24
diets:
  elimination 15–16
  Hay diet 24
  lamb and pear 55

low-sugar 7–12
rotation 15–16, 53–5, 71
vegetarian 50–1, 70–2
digestive system:
  problems 3
  treatment 5–6, 34
dips 46–8, 75–6
dried fruit 8, 17, 19
drinks 23–4

eating:
  in cafés/restaurants 51
  rules for 26–7, 39
Echinacea angustifolia 33
eggs 40, 49, 50, 71
elimination diets 15–16
emotional problems 3
essential fatty acids 34

fat, avoiding 71
fatigue 3
fermented products 20
fibre 39
fibromyalgia 3
fish 21–2, 49, 50, 71, 72
flaxseed oil 34, 40, 42
'foggy' brain syndrome 3
food, left-over 19
food combining 24–6, 50,
    64
food sensitivities/
    intolerances 13–20